How to Improve Your Short-term Memory

Allison C. Lamont PhD & Gillian M. Eadie MEd

Sponsored by:
The Brain and Memory Foundation, New Zealand

How to Improve Your Short-term Memory.
Lamont & Eadie
First Edition, Amazon.

Copyright © 2012 Healthy Memory Company Ltd and authors
Allison Lamont, PhD. & Gillian M. Eadie, MEd.

The moral right of Dr. Allison Lamont and Gillian Eadie to be identified as authors of this work has been asserted in accordance with the Copyright, Designs and Patents Act, 1968. The authors have used their best research endeavours and are not, to their knowledge, infringing any third parties' rights. In the event of queries please contact Healthy Memory Company Limited.

All rights reserved. No part of this book may be used or reproduced in any manner whatsoever without written permission of the authors.

ISBN-13: 978-1477547311
ISBN-10: 1477547312

Published by: Healthy Memory Company Ltd. New Zealand.

Contents

HOW TO PROTECT YOUR MEMORY:	4
PART A: HOW YOUR MEMORY WORKS:	7
What is memory?	15
Why do you forget?	9
PART B: WHAT IS YOUR SHORT-TERM MEMORY?	12
Improve your short-term memory	14
Pay attention	15
Create strong memory traces	15
Exercises	16
Working memory	18
Improve your working memory	18
Memory practice	19
PART C: CREATE YOUR OWN BRAIN FOOD PLAN:	21
Brain boosters you need - shopping list	23
Brain boosting recipe	25
Additional choices to add in following weeks	25
ANSWERS:	26
Memory Tune™	27
OTHER PRODUCTS TO BUILD YOUR BRAIN POWER:	28
APPENDIX:	29
Memory loss or Alzheimer's Disease?	29
Memory problems that aren't part of normal ageing	31
ABOUT THE AUTHORS:	32

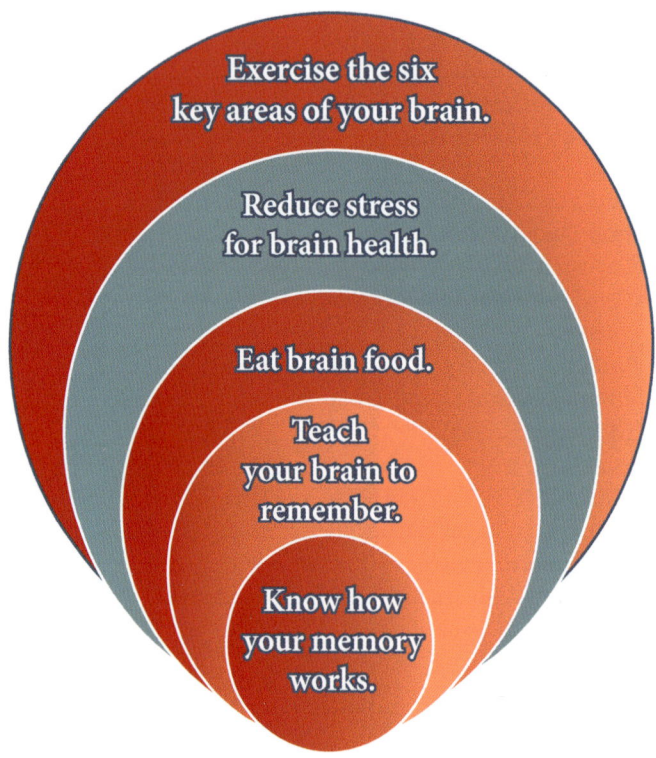

How to Protect Your Memory.©

Do you ....

Forget a name as soon as you hear it?
Go into a room and forget why?
Forget a number when you have just looked it up ?
Have to add numbers again because you lost count?
Fail to recall an address you've just seen on TV!

So, what's happening?

Is this normal?

Are you getting Alzheimer's?[1]

No, your Short-term memory is letting you down.

[1] If you are really worried, turn to pages 29 -31 where the warning signs of dementia are listed. The USA Alzheimer's Foundation suggest memory loss is now the single greatest health worry of baby boomers born between 1946 and 1964

Efficiency in all stages of memory can be improved; short-term memory is just one of the skills you can work on.

The results of actively implementing the memory techniques in this book will surprise you. Not only can you regain lost performance, you can perform better than you did when you were years younger, better than you ever have.

Part A

How your memory works.

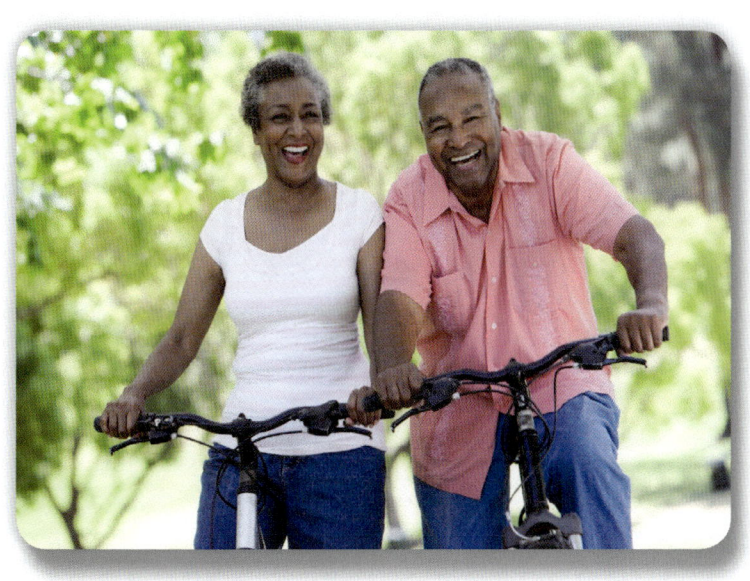

Forgetting things is a normal part of everyday life – at all ages! But not remembering can be extremely embarrassing and inconvenient. The good news is that research shows you can take steps to improve your own memory powers as well as improve your overall brain health.

Everything you know and experience comes to you through the senses of sight, hearing, taste, touch and smell; and that information never stops! You don't need to remember all of it and your brain has efficient ways of sorting out what is important to you. At times, though, your brain needs your help to decide what is important and what isn't.

From the day you are born until the day you die, a healthy brain stores facts, faces, sounds, names, and events along with the emotions that you have connected to them. That's a lot of information! Managing the memory process is quite unconscious until that awful day when you forget something important.

When forgetting occurs more than a few times, there may be a simple explanation e.g. you have been under a lot of stress lately. But it is a wake-up call - a reminder that you cannot take your memory for granted, particularly as you approach your 50's and 60's.

This mini-book focuses on one of the many kinds of memory you can improve: **Short-term Memory**.

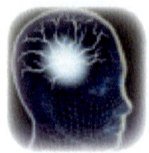

Why do you forget?

Were you paying attention?
Is your brain (and maybe your body) out of shape?
Did you have enough cues or associations?
Has something similar overlaid the details?
Did you understand the information correctly?
Is it a long time since you used the information?
Is stress an issue for you?
Are you sleeping well?
Do you take exercise at least 4 times a week?
Are you on medication?
Is alcohol or substance use an issue for you?

All of these can be factors.

And you can take control of them all!

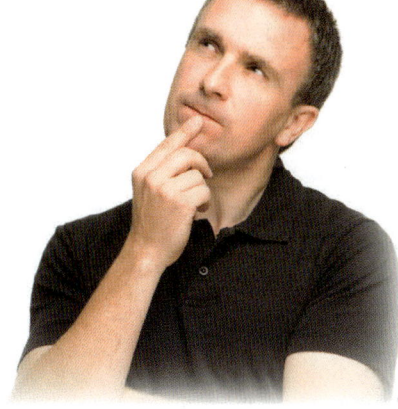

NB: For further information on improving the issues above, see *Seven Second Memory* or *Don't Lose Your Memory! for Busy Executives* by the same authors.

What is Memory?

When you recall an experience or something you have learned previously, you are remembering. For most people, it is impossible to remember everything you experience and it certainly wouldn't be a comfortable experience if you did. Your brain is designed to forget irrelevant details that are not important to you.

Remembering say, a telephone number, involves a complex process as shown in the diagram below.

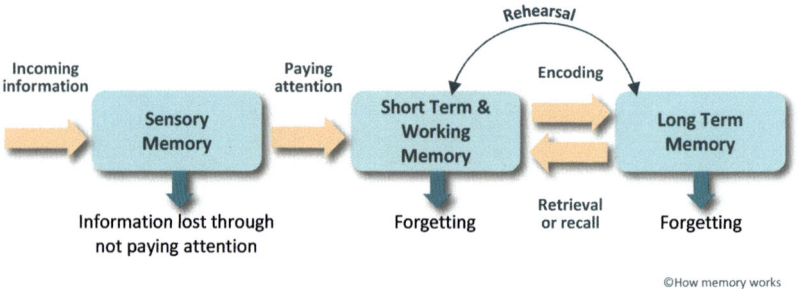

©How memory works

Here's what happens.

You are driving along in the car when you hear an advertisement that interests you with a contact telephone number. There are a lot of other words spoken, music and the sounds of driving. You have to ignore all of those and pay attention to just the telephone number. You might repeat it out loud, or try to 'see' the number in your mind or associate it with another number you already know. It's now in your short-term memory for a few seconds and then, if you have made a sufficiently strong memory trace, it passes into your long-term memory and you will be able to recall it when you get home.

It takes around seven seconds of processing information to create a memory that you will be able to recall later. If you count out seven seconds, you will realize that is quite a long time!

A lot can happen in those seven seconds, though.

If you have to deal with a compulsory stop or traffic lights, your mind may be temporarily distracted. This can enough to interrupt the memory process and the information is lost.

Your brain is really designed to forget so remembering is a miracle!

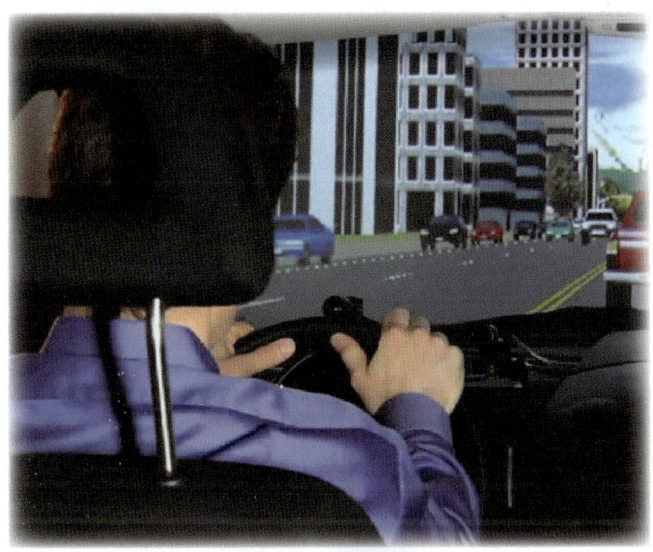

Part B

What is Short-Term Memory?

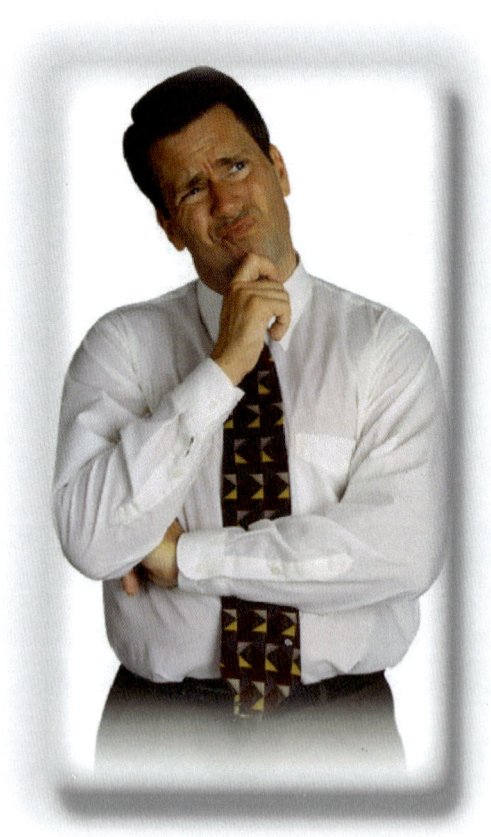

Short-Term Memory

Hearing someone's name then promptly forgetting it, can be embarrassing. That is your short-term memory letting you down.

Bits of information, ideas and thoughts fly in and out of your short-term memory at an amazing rate. And the average person will only retain around seven items (plus or minus 2); and those items will stay with you for only seconds.

The Secret You Need to Know:

To remember any information important to you, **concentration** is needed. It takes **seven seconds of processing** to create a memory trace. Seven seconds! Count it out now - it's a relatively long time. And they need to be seven **active** seconds. Repeating out loud, speaking in rhythm, writing the information down, 'seeing' it in your mind's eye - these will all help create a memory trace and pass into your long-term memory.

Once the information is stored in your long-term memory, it can stay intact for a very long time.

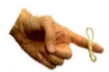

Improve Your Short-term Memory

Short-term memory is a skill that remains with you quite well throughout life, but if you apply some specific techniques, you can make it work even better for you. Often you hear comments such as "His short-term memory is shot! He can't remember what he had for breakfast". This is not actually a short-term memory let-down. It is a recent *long-term memory* lapse. Short-term memory relates to the information you have in your head this very moment.

> *Have you seen the address of a company you want to visit on TV, only to have the details vanish out of your head once the image on the screen disappears? That's short-term memory - it lasts for just a few seconds.*

To master short-term memory, you need to mentally 'shine a light' on the information you want to remember. By repetition out loud, by writing the information down, by going over the address in your mind in a rhythmic way or connecting to a crazy image of your own. These actions create a memory trace that will help process the information into your long-term memory.

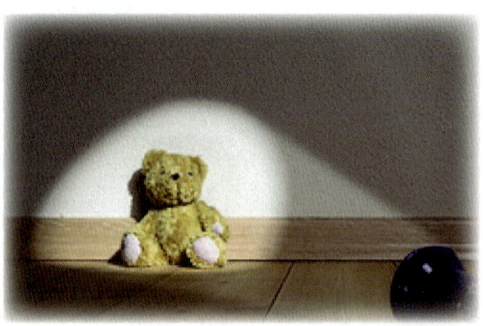

Pay attention!

Focusing on the information you want to remember creates the all important pathway to long-term memory.

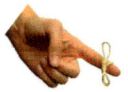

Learn to Create Strong Memory Traces

Take an active interest in establishing positive memory habits. Over-ride auto-pilot for things you particularly want to remember.
Remind yourself of the seven-second rule - it takes seven seconds of concentration to transfer accessible information into your long-term memory.
Pay attention e.g. as the car keys are put down, say aloud, "I'm putting the keys by the phone". Speaking gives you an extra cue.
Use your non-dominant hand to put an item down - using the left hand if you are right-handed is not an automatic action and you are more likely to establish a memory trace to aid recall.
Develop a routine for commonly mislaid items.

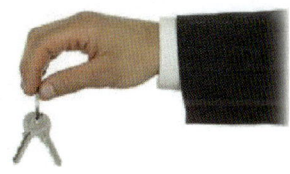

EXERCISE

Knowing that your short-term memory can hold around seven different pieces of information at the same time, you can deliberately practise extending this reach by using the technique of 'chunking' (grouping pieces of information together). For example, read, and try to remember, this sequence of letters:

BBCUSAUKUNGDPIRA

It is a difficult task but, if you chunk them into groups, recall becomes much easier. Try again:

BBC USA UK UN GDP IRA

Practise chunking and retaining information. Try it with a shopping list, for example.

You need:

Jasmine tea, cleaning cloths, dates, dish washing powder, coffee, tomatoes, cranberry juice, furniture polish, blueberries, milk, apples and paper towels.

Close your eyes and try to recall these 12 items.

Did you find this a challenge?

Remembering twelve different items like this while you drive to the supermarket can be made easier.

Chunk the items into three groups (fruit, drinks, cleaning supplies).

This method, which includes the further step of processing the items into the longer term memory, reduces twelve items into three, using each category as a cue for its items. You will now be able to recall the three categories when you reach the supermarket and they, in turn, will evoke the twelve items. Challenge yourself by leaving your shopping list in the car.

(You can always check it before you drive home, just in case. With practice though, you'll find that checking less and less necessary.)

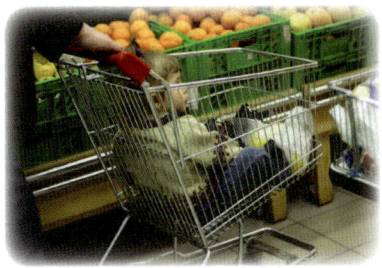

Practise chunking with other items you need to recall: movies you have seen, people who need to be included for a social occasion, tools you need to complete a project, items for the garden and so on.

Your improved short-term memory ability is particularly important for one special type of short-term memory – **working memory.**

Working Memory

Using the seven items of information in your short-term memory to work out an answer or consider options, by trying them out on your 'mental whiteboard', is activating your working memory.

Mental arithmetic at school, or working out the best shopping bargain in a store are everyday examples of your working memory in action.

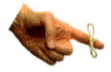

Improve Your Working Memory

1. **Focus on one task at a time.**
2. **Do your most challenging tasks first, while your brain is rested.**
3. **Write down thoughts as they come to you.**
4. **Simplify complicated ideas and concepts.**
5. **Remove distractions.** Turn off mobile alarms!
6. **Remember to Chunk information.**
7. **Feed your working memory.** Keeping a steady supply of glucose and water flowing to your brain is essential. Use fruit and nuts as quick snacks.
8. **Exercise to improve working memory.** A steady supply of oxygen is vital to boost working memory. Blood carries both oxygen and glucose so get those limbs moving!

EXERCISE

Try these:

Write the answer but do the working out 'in your head'.

21 + 84 = ?
769 + 585 = ?
394 + 532 = ?
345 + 456 + 123 = ?
994 + 137 + 376 = ?

Do you know what was happening in the brain during this exercise? You held each step in the calculation in the working memory long enough to find the answer then the details rapidly disappeared.
(Answers on page 27.)

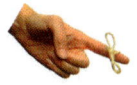

Memory practice for working memory

Wherever you are, you can practise this skill every day. Put aside the calculator for simpler tasks. Mentally calculate the cost of your shopping list or your restaurant order.

Challenge your working memory with Sudoku and crossword puzzles which force you to try out number and word combinations, especially if these are not usual activities for you. Your working memory skills are what others see and judge.

Now you have learned 14 new tips and techniques.

What were they?

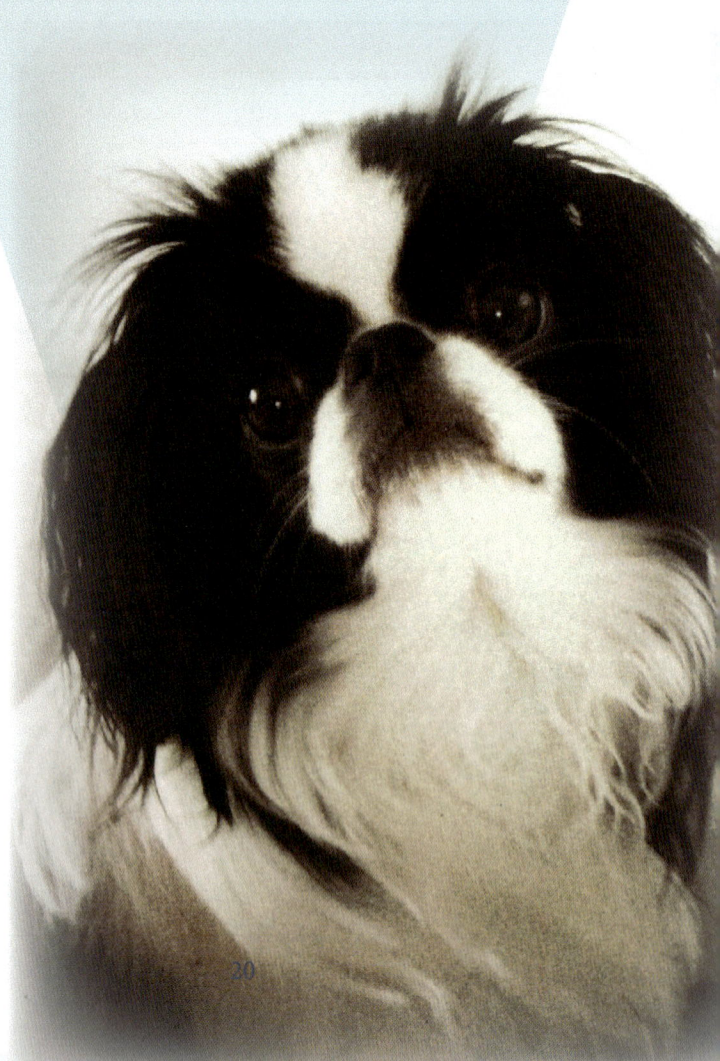

Part C

Create a Brain Food plan.

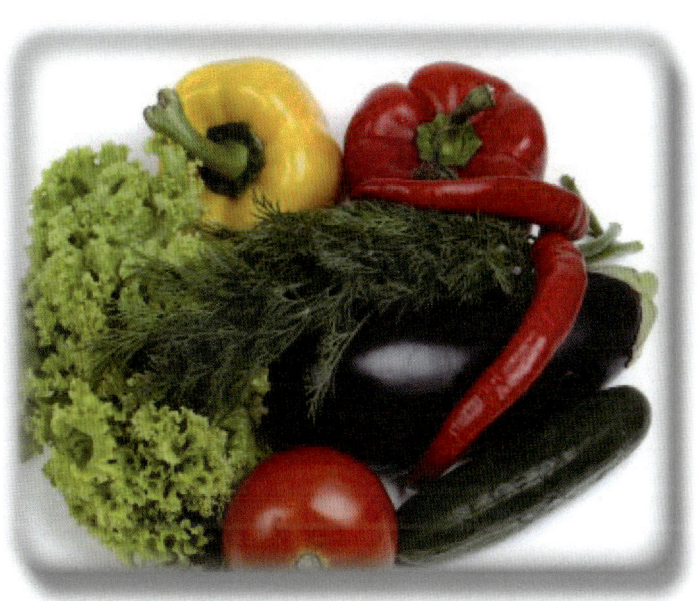

Planning to eat healthily, to support your brain and memory, is an important step in your new way of living.

Five to nine servings of brightly coloured fruits and vegetables a day are recommended. Think about 'eating all the colours of the rainbow'!

Sort out your calorie restricted list of great brain foods to buy and make sure you have plenty of choices to tempt you. Choose around 25 from the list of foods each week. You will find them healthy, low in calories, and covering all of the powerful antioxidants, lean protein, high fibre carbohydrates and good fats that you need.

Your brain-boosting meal plan will guide you over the first few weeks – by then you will be so impressed by the results, you will have your meal planner and lists of foods on the front of your refrigerator!

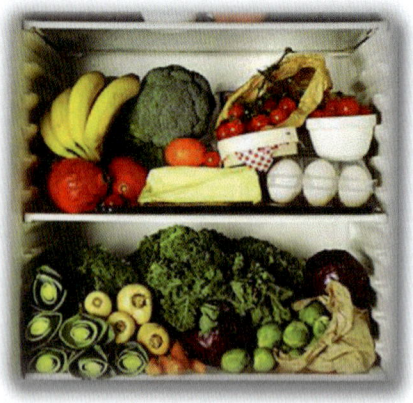

Brain-boosters you need – shopping list

When you are planning your meals for the week, choose around 25 items for your shopping list from the foods are listed below. Each of these is a Brain Food – research has demonstrated that each item has a beneficial effect on your general health, as well as your brain functioning, in particular.

Lean Protein
1. Fish – salmon, tuna, mackerel, herring (also listed under fats)
2. Poultry - chicken and turkey (skinless)
3. Meat - lean beef and pork
4. Eggs – free-range and/or organic eggs are best
5. Tofu and soy products
6. Dairy products - low fat cheeses, cottage cheese, low fat yogurt (sugar free) and low fat or skim milk
7. Beans and lentils - also listed under carbohydrates
8. Nuts and seeds, especially walnuts - also listed under fats

Complex Carbohydrates
1. Berries - especially blueberries, raspberries, strawberries, blackberries (keep frozen berries on hand as well)
2. Oranges, lemons, limes, grapefruit
3. Cherries
4. Peaches, plums
5. Broccoli, cauliflower, brussels sprouts
6. Oats (the long cooking kind), whole wheat items, wholemeal or whole wheat bread with at least 3 grams of fibre.
7. Red or yellow peppers (much higher in Vitamin C than green)
8. Pumpkin squash
9. Spinach – for salad or cooked, adds fibre and nutrients
10. Tomatoes
11. Yams
12. Beans – also listed under proteins

Fats
1. Avocados
2. Extra virgin cold pressed olive oil
3. Olives
4. Salmon - also listed under protein
5. Nuts and nut butter, especially walnuts, macadamia nuts, Brazil nuts, pecans and almonds - also listed under protein

Liquids
1. Water
2. Green or black tea

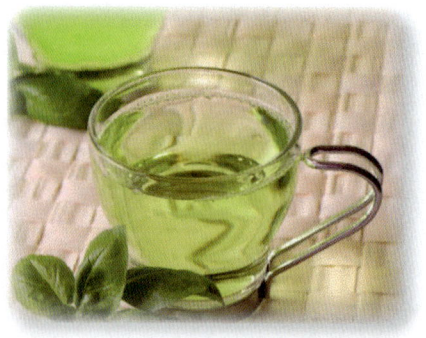

Additional choices to add in following weeks:

Five to nine servings of fruits and vegetables a day are recommended. Have brightly coloured foods on your plate each meal:

red   strawberries, raspberries, cherries, red peppers and tomatoes
yellow squash, yellow peppers, small portions of bananas and peaches
blue   blueberries
purple plums, egg plant (aubergine)
orange oranges, tangerines and yams
green   peas, spinach and broccoli and so on.

It's fun when you begin to think this way and your food looks great on the plate, too.

Brain boosting recipe
Breakfast Smoothie
Handful of frozen berries (or a banana)
Two scoops of protein powder
6 ice cubes
Half a cup of cold milk

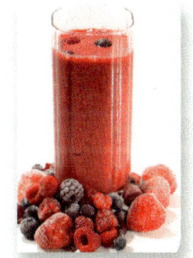

Combine ingredients in blender until smooth.

And that's not all!
There is so much more to know about improving your brain.

If your memory is just out of shape and you feel you are not using your brain effectively enough, the news is good. All kinds of memory can be improved through practice and by using the correct techniques.

In this mini-book, we have covered just one of the important techniques. Short-term memory lapses are the ones most obvious to others, so it is important that you master the techniques for improving this skill.

However, while short-term memory is important, it is not the only memory technique you need. Our advice to you is to follow up with further knowledge and graded practice in the many other critical areas such as verbal and non-verbal memory, prospective memory and face recognition. Lamont & Eadie have two international best-sellers that cover what you need to know (see P. 29).

Memory Tune™ Skills practice delivered to your own computer.

Memory Tune™ a fourteen-part brain and memory training course to improve memory skills in the six key areas.

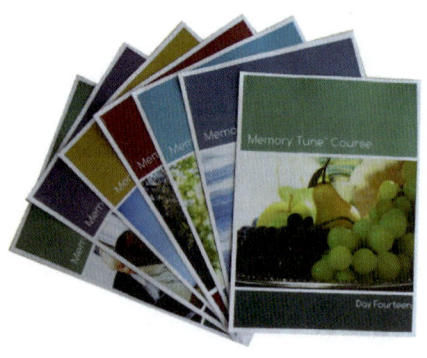

To order: http://brainandmemoryfoundation.org

Efficiency in all stages of memory can be improved; short-term memory is just one of the skills to work on.

An alert and productive memory involves mental agility, nutrition, exercise, rest, paying attention and controlling stress. For many more memory skills, techniques, lifestyle factors and exercises, look for other titles in this series.

You are in control!

Answers

Working memory (page 19)

21 + 84 = (105) 769 + 585 = (1,354)
394 + 532 = (926)
345 + 456 + 123 = (924)
994 + 137 + 376 = (1507)

For more in-depth information about preserving your brain and memory, choose from the following resources.

Authors: Allison Lamont, PhD & Gillian Eadie, MEd, DipTchg.

http://brainandmemoryfoundation.org

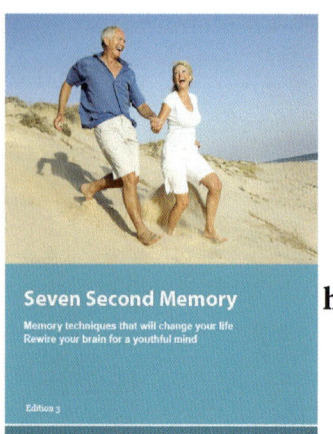

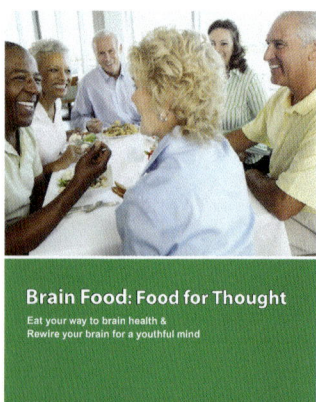

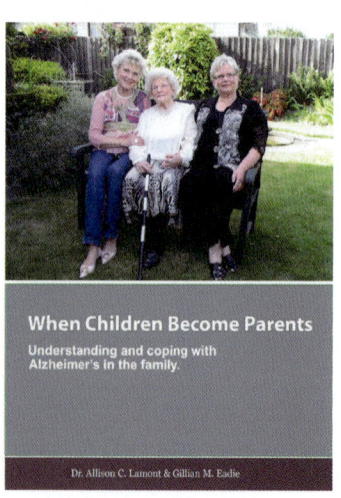

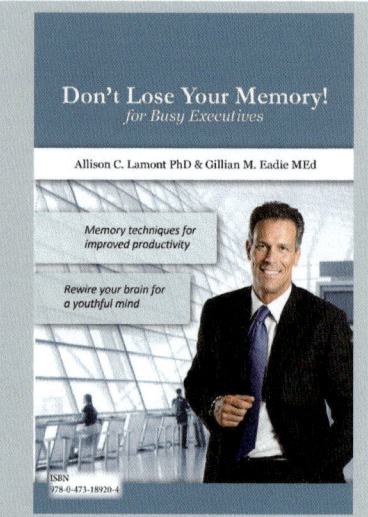

Busy executives have many competing demands on their cognitive abilities. Mid-career, occasional memory lapses can be worrying and detrimental to the professional image needed in business.

'Don't Lose Your Memory!' based on the research findings of Dr. Allison Lamont, provides easily accessible strategies and memory techniques. Advances in knowledge of neuro-plasticity reveal that new brain connections can be developed at any age. This reassuring news makes the few minutes a day of self-investment imperative for mature executives. This exciting new handbook will show how.

APPENDIX

Memory loss or Alzheimer's Disease?

An everyday memory lapse such as a tip-of-the-tongue lapse or not being able to recall a friend's name often raises fears of dementia. Dementias are brain disorders that seriously affect a person's ability to carry out daily activities. The most common cause of dementia is Alzheimer's Disease.

While a problem with memory is an early symptom of Alzheimer's and other dementias, both the symptoms and the underlying biological brain changes are very different to those of normal memory loss which may occur with ageing. Dementia involves a broad loss of cognitive and intellectual abilities, only one of which is memory. For example, forgetting where you put your glasses can happen to everyone occasionally, but forgetting you need glasses at all may be a cause for concern.

Dementia is a medical condition which causes disruption in the way the brain works, bringing with it impaired cognitive functioning on a wide range of abilities, particularly thought, memory, and language. Dementia can affect people at any age, and it is not part of the normal ageing process.

The number of people being diagnosed with Alzheimer's, a neurodegenerative disease, is growing because people are living longer than in earlier times.

Scientific investigation continues into the causes of dementia, where brain neurons (brain cells) deteriorate and eventually lose function. Investigators generally agree that an abnormally increased development of amyloid plaques (a sticky protein) and neurofibrillary tangles, is a defining characteristic of Alzheimer's. Brain-imaging studies have also shown that those with Alzheimer's have a smaller hippocampus (the structure deep in the brain, vital to the formation of memories) than healthy people, and consistently show damage to the brain pathways that link the hippocampus to the other brain areas necessary to cognitive functioning.

Besides memory problems, one of the early signs of Alzheimer's in some people is difficulty with language and routine activities such as shopping or driving. Hallmarks of Alzheimer's are mood and behavioural changes, and outbursts of aggression, delusions, agitation, and verbal abusiveness. Daily tasks such as dressing, showering, or making a cup of tea may be compromised.

Recent studies, however, have found that some people live into advanced old age with little memory loss even though, after death, their brains show damage from Alzheimer's disease. It is important to remember that Alzheimer's is not part of normal ageing. Research suggests that keeping mentally engaged and physically active builds the strongest protection against the symptoms of Alzheimer's. This resilience is known as brain plasticity.

Memory problems that aren't part of normal ageing

- Forgetting autobiographical information
- Having trouble learning new things
- Profound difficulty in recalling objects, places, times, dates, names
- Forgetting how to do everyday tasks you've done many times before
- Not recognizing family or friends
- Forgetting how to maintain personal hygiene
- Repeating phrases or stories in the same conversation
- Trouble making choices or handling money
- Unable to find your way in familiar surroundings
- Tendency to wander aimlessly from your home
- Noticeable language and intellectual decline
- Poor judgement
- A growing sense of distrust
- Unusual irritability and/or aggressiveness
- Noticeable change of personality in later stages of the disease
- Inability to keep track of day to day events
- General loss of social graces
- Inability to follow simple instructions or concentrate
- Feeling more depressed, confused, restless and anxious
- Delusions or hallucinations

If you believe you, or someone close to you, may be developing Alzheimer's, ask your general practitioner to refer you to a neurologist or a neuropsychologist who will carry out diagnostic tests and provide advice on how best to cope with the life difficulties which accompanies dementia.

About the Authors:

The two authors established the Healthy Memory Company in 2008. Their articles, books and memory programmes are scientifically based on Dr. Lamont's research findings and focus on the key skills needed to keep brains active, alert and growing at any age. For most people, brain skills are still intact at age 50 and this is when it is best to begin developing the cognitive reserve that will maintain productivity and buffer the brain against memory loss later in life. Gillian and Allison are executive baby boomers themselves and regularly address groups nationally and at international conferences.

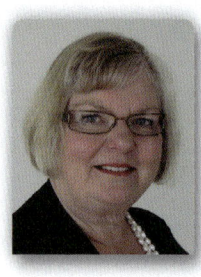

Dr. Allison C. Lamont, PhD, MA (First Class Honours) MNZAC, MNZPsS, MAPS. Dr. Lamont's ground-breaking research into memory in older, healthy adults has excited interest in many parts of the world. She has addressed audiences in USA, the UK and New Zealand. Published by Verlag, Germany her research is on sale in bookstores and through Amazon.com. Allison has her own counselling practice and Memory Clinic in New Zealand. http://memoryclinic.co.nz

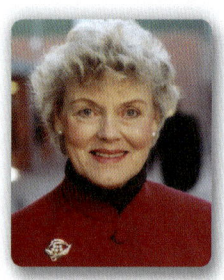

Gillian M. Eadie, M.Ed, BA, Dip.Tchg, LTCL, Churchill Fellow, HFNZCS, Churchill Millennium Fellow. Gillian is an award-winning educator and speech pathologist whose career includes 20 years as principal in prestigious private schools. She manages the Confucius Institute and chaired the Ethics Committee at The University of Auckland, New Zealand.

Other books in the series include:
Brain Food: Food for Thought, Edition 3
Seven Second Memory. Memory techniques that will change your life Ed.3
When Children Become Parents: A guide to understanding and coping with Alzheimer's in your family.
Don't Lose Your Memory! for Busy Executives. New

See also **Memory Tune™** - a fourteen-part brain training course to improve memory skills in the six key areas for independence in older age.

Visit http://brainandmemoryfoundation.org/product for purchases.

Disclaimer

All materials in this publication including but not limited to photographs, logos, text, sounds, music, layout configuration, source code is the subject of copyright in general owned by Healthy Memory Company Ltd. unless otherwise acknowledged. No unauthorized copying of any of this material is permitted. For authorisation to reproduce anything in this book please contact us.

Use and browsing of this book or our site is at your own risk. If you are dissatisfied with any of the materials contained in the book, or Site or with anything in these Terms of Use, your sole remedy is to discontinue accessing and using the book or Site.

To the fullest extent permissible under applicable law, neither Healthy Memory Company Ltd. nor any other party involved in creating, producing or delivering this book is liable for any direct, incidental, consequential, indirect or punitive damages arising out of your access to, or use of, the book or Site. Without limiting the foregoing, everything in the book or Site is provided to you "as is" without warranty of any kind, either expressed or implied, including, but not limited to, the accuracy of any information, the implied warranties or merchantability, fitness for a particular purpose, or non-infringement of any product or service. In particular, the information contained in this book or on this site should not be taken as medical advice. Medical advances and practices can be complex and can change without warning. We do not guarantee the accuracy of any information in this book as it applies to you at any particular time or for any particular purpose. Before relying on any information you should seek specific advice from your doctor.

You specifically acknowledge and agree that Healthy Memory Company Ltd. is not liable for any defamatory, offensive or illegal conduct of any user of the blogs, forum or other messaging relating to the book or Site.

Healthy Memory Company Ltd. also assumes no responsibility, and shall not be liable for any damages to, or viruses that may infect, your computer equipment or other property on account of your access to, use of, or browsing of the book or Site (including any Bulletin Board) or your downloading of any Materials from the Site.

Healthy Memory Company Ltd. does not warrant or make any representations of any kind or nature with respect to the Materials in this book or on this Site. Therefore, you are responsible for compliance with local laws, if and to the extent local laws are applicable.

Personal information obtained by Healthy Memory Company Ltd. through the use of this book or Site will not be disclosed to third parties.

In the event of queries, please contact Healthy Memory Company Limited.
   editor@healthymemorycompany.com

Printed in Great Britain
by Amazon.co.uk, Ltd.,
Marston Gate.